The Core Transformation Challenge

Master the Russian Twist and See Results

Helen Talbott

Disclaimer:

The information and exercises presented in this book are intended for general informational purposes only and should not be interpreted as medical, nutritional, or professional fitness advice. Always consult with a qualified healthcare professional, licensed dietitian, or certified personal trainer before starting any new exercise program, especially if you have any pre-existing medical conditions, injuries, or limitations. They can assess your individual needs and design a safe and effective workout plan tailored to your specific circumstances.

Individual Results May Vary:

The exercises and program presented in this book are not guaranteed to produce specific results for everyone. Individual responses to exercise are highly variable and depend on factors such as genetics, fitness level, nutrition, and overall health. Do not compare your progress to others; focus on your own journey and celebrate your personal achievements.

Assumption of Risk:

By participating in the exercises and program outlined in this book, you acknowledge and assume the inherent risks associated with physical activity. It is your responsibility to exercise caution, modify exercises as needed, and stop if you experience any pain or discomfort.

Limitation of Liability:

The author and publisher are not liable for any injuries, losses, or damages incurred as a result of using the information contained within this book. It is your responsibility to use this information safely and responsibly.

Copyright and Intellectual Property:

The content of this book is protected by copyright and intellectual property laws. Copying, reproducing, or distributing any portion of this book without the express written permission of the author is strictly prohibited.

Affiliate Disclosures:

Some information contained within this book may mention or link to products or services offered by the author, affiliates, or partners. However, any such mentions or links are for informational purposes only and do not constitute endorsements or recommendations. It is your responsibility to conduct your own research and due diligence before making any purchases.

Final Note:

We encourage you to approach your core transformation journey with enthusiasm, knowledge, and a healthy dose of caution. Always prioritize your safety and well-being, and remember that a strong core is just one piece of a healthy and fulfilling life.

Table of contents

About the author

I'm Helen Talbott and my passion lies at the intersection of fitness, empowerment, and helping individuals unlock their full potential. As a certified personal trainer, fitness enthusiast, health advocate, I've witnessed firsthand the transformative power of core strength, both physically and mentally.

My journey with the Russian Twist wasn't simply about mastering an exercise; it was about discovering its potential to unlock deeper strength, resilience, and self-belief. This realization fueled my desire to share this transformative experience with others, leading me to create "The Core Transformation Challenge: Master the Russian Twist and See Results."

In this book, I draw upon my knowledge, experience, and enthusiasm to guide you through a **structured yet adaptable challenge**. By mastering the Russian Twist and exploring its variations, you'll not only sculpt a stronger core but also cultivate discipline, confidence, and a deeper connection to your physical potential.

But my writing goes beyond mere instruction. I believe in creating a supportive community where individuals can learn, share, and motivate each other. That's why you'll find within these pages:

- **Personal anecdotes and experiences:** I share my own journey with the Russian Twist, offering relatable and inspiring insights.
- **Science-backed information:** The benefits of core strength and the effectiveness of the Russian Twist are grounded in evidence, which I present in a clear and engaging way.
- **Motivational guidance:** I understand the challenges and triumphs of any fitness journey, and I offer encouragement and support throughout the book.
- **A holistic approach:** Building a strong core isn't just about aesthetics; it's about overall well-being. I emphasize the

importance of proper nutrition, rest, and recovery for lasting results.

"The Core Transformation Challenge" is more than just a book; it's an invitation to **join a movement** of individuals who believe in the transformative power of core strength. By empowering your core, you empower yourself to live a healthier, happier, and more confident life.

Connect with me to:

- Share your progress and challenges.
- Get inspired by other participants.
- Ask questions and receive support.

Let's embark on this transformative journey together. Remember, a strong core is not just about physical strength; it's about building the strength to achieve your goals and embrace life with confidence.

Start your transformation today!

Introduction

Welcome to the Core Transformation Challenge!

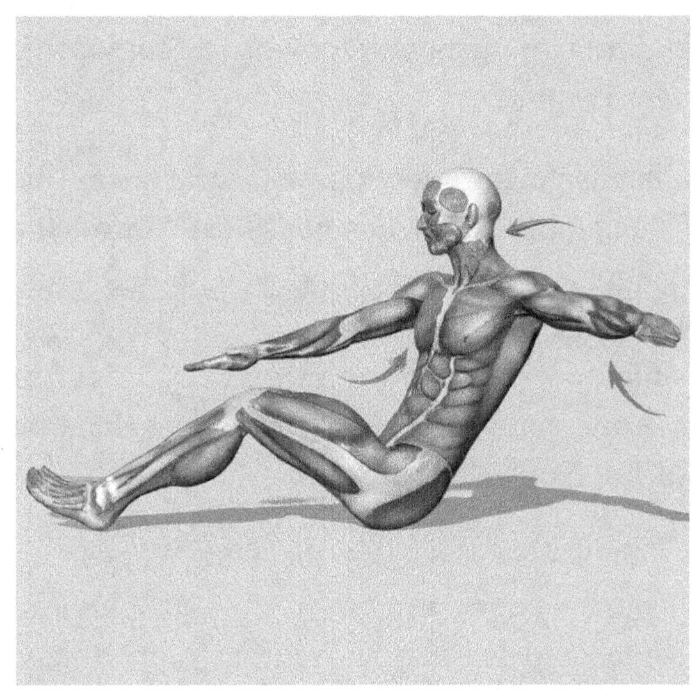

Are you ready to **unlock a stronger, more defined core**? Are you tired of crunches and sit-ups delivering underwhelming results? Then prepare to be **twisted** - in the best way possible!

This is not your average "fitness book." No fad diets, no fancy equipment, just pure, unadulterated **core-crushing intensity** with the **Russian Twist** as your weapon. This ancient exercise, rooted in martial arts, has been passed down through generations for a reason: it **delivers results**.

This intensive introduction will strip away the fluff and **thrust you headfirst into the challenge**. Forget everything you thought you knew about core training. Here, we're not messing around. We're **targeting every layer of your core**, building **stability, strength, and definition** like never before.

This challenge is not for the faint of heart. It will **push your limits**, test your **mental fortitude**, and leave you wanting more (okay, maybe sometimes less, but trust me, the results are worth it!).

Are you ready to:

- **Feel the burn** like never before?

- **See your abs start to peek through** in just weeks?
- **Boost your metabolism** and **improve your overall fitness**?
- **Join a community of challengers** pushing each other to the finish line?

If you answered **YES** to any of these questions, then **strap yourself in!** The **Core Transformation Challenge:** with the **Russian Twist** is about to change the way you see core training, and your body, forever.

Ready to embark on this transformative journey? Turn the page and let's begin!

Setting Fire to Your Core: Goals, Expectations, and the Twist Within

Before you embark on this transformative journey, let's talk about **goals and expectations**. This isn't a walk in the park (or a leisurely stroll on the yoga mat). The **Russian Twist Challenge** demands commitment, but the rewards are substantial. To navigate this intense adventure successfully, **setting clear goals and realistic expectations** is crucial.

Goal Setting: Beyond Rock-Hard Abs

Sure, washboard abs might be the ultimate visual reward, but let's **dig deeper**. What truly motivates you? Is it:

- **Improved athletic performance?** Do you dream of hitting harder, throwing farther, or running faster?
- **Pain-free movement?** Are you tired of backaches hindering your activities?
- **Increased confidence and strength?** Do you desire a stronger, more capable body that reflects your inner fire?

Identifying your **"why"** will fuel your motivation throughout the challenge. Once you know your core (pun intended) desire, translate it into **SMART goals**:

- **Specific:** Instead of "get fit," aim for "do 20 uninterrupted Russian Twists with weights by week 4."

- **Measurable:** Track your progress by reps, sets, weights, or even how your clothes fit.
- **Attainable:** Don't set yourself up for failure. Start with achievable goals and gradually progress.
- **Relevant:** Ensure your goals align with your "why" and overall fitness aspirations.
- **Time-bound:** Give yourself a deadline to stay accountable.

Expectation Check: Embrace the Journey, Not Just the Finish Line

This challenge is **intense**. Setbacks, soreness, and moments of doubt are inevitable. Here's how to keep your expectations realistic:

- **Focus on progress, not perfection:** It's a journey, not a sprint. Celebrate small wins and acknowledge your dedication.
- **Listen to your body:** Rest when needed. Pushing through pain can lead to injury.
- **Embrace the community:** Support from fellow challengers can be invaluable.

Share your struggles and celebrate victories together.

- **Enjoy the process:** Find exercises you enjoy, and don't be afraid to modify!

Remember, this challenge is about **transformation, not just reaching a specific endpoint**. Enjoy the process of **discovering a stronger, more capable you**. Embrace the burn, celebrate the twist, and watch your core transform along the way!

Now, are you ready to set your goals and conquer the Russian Twist? Turn the page and ignite your core transformation!

The best part about the **Russian Twist Challenge** is that it requires **minimal equipment**, making it accessible to everyone, anywhere! Here's what you might need, but remember, most variations can be done with just your bodyweight:

Essentials:

- **Comfy workout clothes:** Opt for breathable fabrics that allow for unrestricted movement.
- **Exercise mat (optional):** Provides cushioning and grip, especially on hard surfaces.
- **Water bottle:** Stay hydrated before, during, and after your workouts.

Optional Equipment (for added challenge):

- **Medicine ball:** Choose a weight that allows you to maintain proper form with controlled twists.

- **Dumbbells:** Similar to medicine balls, choose a weight that challenges without compromising form.
- **Weight plate:** If you have access to weight plates, they can also be used for weighted twists.
- **Towel (optional):** Can be placed under your lower back for added comfort and support.

Remember:

- Start with bodyweight variations and gradually progress to using weights as your core strengthens.
- Choose equipment that feels comfortable and allows you to maintain proper form throughout the exercises.
- Listen to your body and adjust the weight or difficulty as needed.
- Focus on quality over quantity when adding weights.

No matter what equipment you choose, the key is to commit to the challenge and embrace the power of the Russian Twist!

Chapter 1

Unveiling the Core: Anatomy and Biomechanics of the Russian Twist

The **Russian Twist** might seem like a simple twist of the torso, but beneath the surface lies a complex interplay of muscles and mechanics. Understanding this dance of anatomy and biomechanics is crucial for maximizing the effectiveness of your workouts and avoiding injury. So, buckle up and let's delve into the core of the matter!

Meet Your Core Crew:

The **Russian Twist** primarily targets your **obliques**, the powerhouse muscles located on the sides of your torso. These deep abdominal muscles work in conjunction with your:

- **Rectus abdominis:** The "six-pack" muscle at the front of your abdomen,

providing stability and assisting with
rotation.

- **Transverse abdominis:** Your deepest
core muscle, like a natural corset, helping
maintain spinal stability and
intra-abdominal pressure.
- **Lower back muscles:** They work
synergistically with the core to ensure
proper form and prevent excessive strain
on the spine.

The Twisting Symphony:

When you perform the **Russian Twist**, imagine
your core muscles like an orchestra:

- **Obliques:** Lead the melody, providing the
primary twisting force and rotational
power.
- **Rectus abdominis:** Harmonizes with the
obliques, adding stability and contributing
to the twist.
- **Transverse abdominis:** Acts like the
conductor, ensuring everything works

together smoothly and maintaining core tension.

- **Lower back muscles:** Play a supporting role, keeping your spine in alignment and preventing unwanted arching.

Biomechanics in Action:

As you twist, your obliques contract on one side while lengthening on the other, generating rotational force. This force works against the resistance of your bodyweight or added weight, creating a challenging exercise that strengthens your core muscles.

Beyond the Obvious:

While the **Russian Twist** primarily targets your core, it also indirectly engages other muscle groups:

- **Shoulders:** Stabilize your upper body and help you maintain proper form.
- **Hips and glutes:** Contribute to torso stability and prevent excessive movement in the lower body.

- **Legs:** Maintain balance and provide resistance when you lower your legs towards the ground.

Understanding these biomechanical principles allows you to:

- **Optimize your form:** Target the right muscles with proper technique, maximizing results and minimizing injury risk.
- **Progress effectively:** Choose variations and progressions that challenge your core muscles in different ways.
- **Listen to your body:** Identify potential imbalances or weaknesses and adjust your workouts accordingly.

Ready to turn theory into practice? The next chapter dives deep into proper form and technique, ensuring you unlock the full potential of this core-crushing exercise!

Chapter 2

Mastering the Twist: Step-by-Step Guide to Perfect Form

Now that you understand the anatomy and biomechanics of the **Russian Twist**, it's time to transform knowledge into action. This chapter guides you through mastering proper form and technique, ensuring you unleash the **full core-crushing potential** of this exercise. Remember, proper form is your armor against injury and your key to maximizing results.

Gearing Up for the Twist:

1. **Find your battleground:** Choose a comfortable yet firm surface like an exercise mat or carpeted floor.
2. **Prepare your posture:** Stand tall with your feet hip-width apart, engaging your core by pulling your belly button towards your spine.

3. **Initiate the descent:** Lean back slightly, forming a 45-degree angle with your torso and the ground. Keep your spine straight and core engaged.
4. **Raise the shield:** Extend your arms straight out in front of you, palms facing inward, or interlace your fingers for added stability.

The Twisting Dance:

1. **Engage, rotate, control:** Exhale as you rotate your torso to one side, leading with your core, not your arms. Feel the tension in your obliques as you turn.
2. **Slow and steady wins the race:** Avoid jerky movements. Aim for a controlled twist, focusing on engaging your core throughout the entire range of motion.
3. **Touchdown, but keep flying:** Don't let your hips touch the ground. Maintain a slight hover, creating tension in your core and challenging your stability.
4. **The return voyage:** Inhale as you twist back to the center, feeling the opposite

oblique engage. Don't rush; maintain
control and proper form.

5. **Repeat and conquer:** Continue twisting
   to the other side, completing the same
   controlled movement. Aim for a desired
   number of repetitions or sets.

Form Check: Your Core's Guardian Angel:

- **Keep your back straight:** Avoid
  hunching or arching your spine.
  Maintaining a neutral spine is crucial for
  preventing injury.
- **Core engaged, not inflated:** Don't puff
  out your chest. Draw your belly button in
  and keep your core tight throughout the
  movement.
- **Eyes on the horizon:** Avoid looking
  down as you twist. Keep your gaze
  forward or slightly upward to maintain
  neck alignment.
- **Breath your way through:** Exhale as you
  twist and inhale as you return to center.
  Breathing helps maintain core tension and
  control.

- **Don't force it:** If you feel pain, stop and adjust your form or weight.

Remember: Form is paramount. It might feel slower at first, but focusing on proper technique will yield better results and keep you safe throughout your core transformation challenge.

Mastering the basics is just the beginning. The next chapter unlocks exciting variations and progressions, taking your core challenge to the next level!

Chapter 3

Twisting Up the Challenge: Variations & Progressions for Core Domination

Ready to push your limits and explore the diverse world of the **Russian Twist**? This chapter unveils a treasure trove of variations and progressions, catering to all levels of fitness and adding spice to your core workouts. Dive in and discover the perfect twist for you!

Level Up Your Core Game:

Beginner:

- **Kneeling Twist:** Start by kneeling instead of leaning back, reducing intensity and focusing on form.

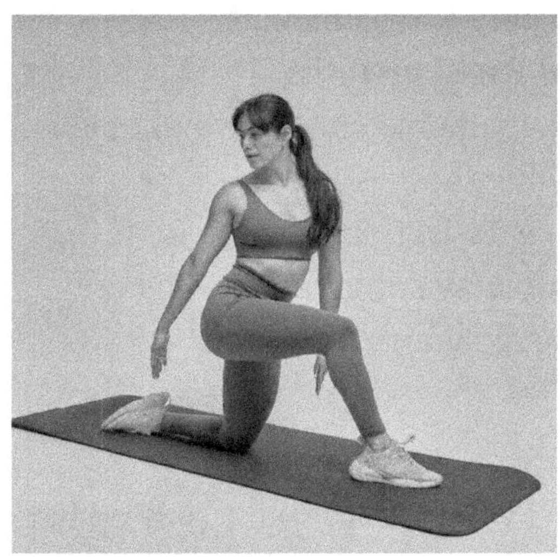

- **Assisted Twist:** Use a stable object like a chair or wall for support as you lean back and twist.

- **Weighted Kneeling Twist:** Once comfortable, hold a light weight (water bottle, book) close to your chest for added challenge.

Intermediate:

- **Full Plank Twist:** Progress to a full plank position with forearms on the ground for increased core engagement.
- **Weighted Russian Twist:** Hold a dumbbell, medicine ball, or weight plate close to your chest as you twist.
- **Single-Leg Twist:** Raise one leg off the ground while twisting, increasing core stability and balance.

Advanced:

- **Hanging Twist:** Hang from a pull-up bar and perform controlled twists, challenging your grip and core strength.
- **Anti-Rotation Twist:** Hold a medicine ball or weight to one side and resist rotation, mimicking real-world athletic movements.

- **Weighted Plate Twist:** Hold a weight plate behind your head for even greater core and shoulder engagement.

Bonus Twists:

- **Medicine Ball Slam Twist:** Add a medicine ball slam in between twists for an explosive core and upper body workout.
- **Russian Twist with Leg Raise:** Simultaneously raise one leg as you twist, further challenging your core and stability.
- **Partner Twist:** Perform the twist with a partner, passing a medicine ball for an interactive and dynamic core challenge.

Remember:

- Start with easier variations and progress gradually to avoid injury.
- Choose variations that target your specific fitness goals and weaknesses.
- Listen to your body and adjust the weight, intensity, or variation as needed.

- Don't forget to have fun! Experiment and find variations you enjoy to keep your workouts engaging.

This is just a taste of the endless possibilities the Russian Twist offers. With these variations and progressions, you can design personalized workouts that keep your core challenged, engaged, and sculpted throughout your transformation journey!

Ready to put your core to the test? The next chapter equips you with essential safety tips and precautions to ensure you dominate the challenge injury-free!

Chapter 4

Twisting Safely: Avoiding Common Mistakes on Your Core Transformation Journey

The **Russian Twist** is a powerful exercise, but improper form or technique can lead to injury. This chapter equips you with the knowledge to identify and avoid common mistakes, ensuring you **conquer the challenge safely and effectively**.

Mistake #1: Sacrificing Form for Speed:

It's tempting to rush through repetitions, but remember, **quality over quantity**. Maintain controlled movements, focusing on engaging your core throughout the entire range of motion. Avoid jerky motions that put undue stress on your spine.

Mistake #2: Hunching Your Back:

Keep your spine **neutral and straight**, avoiding rounding your shoulders or arching your lower back. This protects your spine and ensures your core muscles are working optimally.

Mistake #3: Letting Your Hips Touch Down:

Maintaining a slight hover keeps your **core engaged and challenged**. Letting your hips touch the ground reduces core tension and defeats the purpose of the exercise.

Mistake #4: Twisting with Your Arms:

Your core, not your arms, should initiate the twist. **Use your arms for balance**, not momentum. Avoid swinging your arms back and forth, as this reduces core engagement.

Mistake #5: Going Too Heavy, Too Soon:

Start with your bodyweight and gradually progress to weights. Using weights that are too heavy compromises form and increases the risk of injury. **Focus on proper form before adding weight.**

Mistake #6: Ignoring Pain:

Don't push through pain. If you feel discomfort, stop and adjust your form, weight, or variation. Ignoring pain can lead to serious injuries.

Mistake #7: Neglecting Warm-up and Cool-down:

Prepare your body for the challenge with a **dynamic warm-up** and end with a **static cool-down**. This helps prevent injuries and improves muscle recovery.

Mistake #8: Neglecting Rest and Recovery:

Give your body time to rebuild and repair. Make sure to **schedule rest days** and incorporate **recovery strategies** like stretching and foam rolling.

Mistake #9: Comparing Yourself to Others:

Everyone progresses at their own pace. **Focus on your own journey** and celebrate your personal achievements.

Mistake #10: Giving Up:

Challenges are meant to be challenging! There will be tough days, but remember **your goals and why you started**. Stay motivated, adapt your workouts, and celebrate small wins along the way.

By understanding and avoiding these common mistakes, you can maximize the effectiveness of your Russian Twist Challenge and achieve your core transformation goals, safely and successfully!

Next up, dive into the core of your challenge with the weekly workout plans, ready to ignite your core transformation!

Chapter 5

Embark on Your Transformation: The 4-Week Challenge Structure

Welcome to the heart of your core transformation journey! This chapter unveils the **4-week challenge structure**, your roadmap to sculpted abs and a stronger, more defined core. Get ready to be challenged, motivated, and inspired as you unlock your true potential with the **Russian Twist**.

The Core of the Challenge:

- **Duration:** 4 weeks, progressively building in intensity and difficulty.
- **Frequency:** 3 workouts per week, allowing adequate rest and recovery.
- **Structure:** Each workout focuses on different core variations and progressions, keeping your core engaged and challenged.

- **Flexibility:** Modifications and alternate exercises are provided to cater to different fitness levels and abilities.
- **Community:** Optional access to a supportive online community for motivation, tips, and shared experiences (consider adding details on how to access this community).

Weekly Progression:

Each week follows a specific theme, gradually increasing intensity and complexity:

- **Week 1: Mastering the Basics:** Focus on proper form and technique with bodyweight variations.
- **Week 2: Building Strength:** Introduce weighted variations and progressions to challenge your core further.
- **Week 3: Pushing Limits:** Explore advanced variations and combinations for an intense core workout.

- **Week 4: Peak Performance:** Fine-tune your form and challenge yourself with peak variations to optimize results.

Remember:

- Listen to your body and take rest days when needed.
- Don't be afraid to modify exercises or weights to match your fitness level.
- Track your progress to stay motivated and celebrate your achievements.
- Enjoy the journey! Embrace the challenge and experience the transformative power of the Russian Twist.

Ready to delve into the specific workout plans? Buckle up, because the next chapters unlock the weekly blueprints for your core domination!

Important Note: You might want to include a brief summary of each week's theme and key exercises in this chapter to create a sense of anticipation and excitement for the reader. This

would also provide a high-level overview of the
challenge structure before diving into the details
of each week's plan.

Week 1: Mastering the Basics - Ignite Your Core!

Welcome to Week 1! This is your foundation week, where you'll solidify your technique and build a strong base for the core-crushing adventures ahead. Remember, **form is paramount**, so prioritize quality over quantity and listen to your body. Let's ignite your core!

Key Focus:

- Mastering proper form and technique for the **Russian Twist** and its variations.
- Building core strength and endurance with foundational exercises.
- Establishing a consistent workout routine and listening to your body.

Workout Structure:

This week features three 30-minute workouts, each focusing on different aspects of core training. You can perform them on alternate days, allowing rest and recovery for maximum results.

Workout 1: Core Fundamentals:

- **Warm-up:** 5 minutes of light cardio (jumping jacks, jogging in place) and dynamic stretches (arm circles, torso twists).
- **Russian Twist (bodyweight):** 3 sets of 10-12 repetitions per side. Focus on controlled movements and core engagement.
- **Plank:** 3 sets of 30-second holds. Modify on knees if needed.
- **Bird-Dog:** 3 sets of 10 repetitions per side. Engage your core and maintain a neutral spine.
- **Dead Bug:** 3 sets of 15 repetitions. Control the movement and keep your lower back pressed to the ground.
- **Cool-down:** 5 minutes of static stretches focusing on your core, back, and legs.

Workout 2: Stability Challenge:

- **Warm-up:** Same as Workout 1.

- **Side Plank with Reach-Through:** 3 sets of 10-12 repetitions per side. Engage your core and maintain a straight line from head to heel.
- **Anti-Rotation Press:** 3 sets of 10-12 repetitions per side. Hold a light weight and resist rotation while pressing overhead.
- **Single-Leg Romanian Deadlift:** 3 sets of 10-12 repetitions per leg. Maintain a flat back and keep your core engaged.
- **Hollow Body Hold:** 3 sets of 30-second holds. Press your lower back to the ground and focus on core engagement.
- **Cool-down:** Same as Workout 1.

Workout 3: Core Activation Blast:

- **Warm-up:** Same as Workout 1.
- **Walking Russian Twist:** 3 sets of 15 repetitions per side. Walk your hands to one side, perform a twist, and walk back to the center.
- **Mountain Climbers:** 3 sets of 30 seconds. Maintain a high plank position

and alternate bringing your knees towards
your chest.

- **Plank Hip Twists:** 3 sets of 10 repetitions per side. In a plank position, rotate your hips from side to side while keeping your core engaged.
- **Side Plank Leg Raises:** 3 sets of 10-12 repetitions per side. Raise your top leg while maintaining a side plank position.
- **Cool-down:** Same as Workout 1.

Remember:

- Modify exercises as needed. It's better to do them correctly with bodyweight than risk injury with weights.
- Track your progress! Note down reps, sets, and any modifications you make.
- Stay hydrated and fuel your body with healthy foods for optimal results.
- Join the community (if available) and share your experiences with fellow challengers!

Congratulations on completing Week 1! You've laid the foundation for a strong core. Get ready to push your limits and unleash your inner core warrior in Week 2!

Week 2: Building Strength - Unleash Your Core Power!

Week 1 laid the groundwork, and now it's time to **crank up the intensity**! This week focuses on **building strength and endurance** with weighted variations and progressions. Embrace the burn, feel your core ignite, and prepare to witness its transformation.

Key Focus:

- Introducing weighted variations of the Russian Twist and other core exercises.
- Increasing reps, sets, or adding weights to challenge your core further.
- Maintaining proper form while pushing your limits.

Workout Structure:

Similar to Week 1, you'll have three 30-minute workouts focusing on different aspects of core training. Remember to rest when needed and prioritize proper form over heavier weights.

Workout 1: Weighted Core Challenge:

- **Warm-up:** Same as Week 1.
- **Weighted Russian Twist:** 3 sets of 8-10 repetitions per side with light weights (medicine ball, dumbbell). Focus on controlled movements and core engagement.
- **Weighted Plank:** 3 sets of 30-second holds with weights on your back (backpack, sandbag).
- **Kneeling Anti-Rotation Chop:** 3 sets of 10-12 repetitions per side with medicine ball or light weight. Engage your core and resist rotation.
- **Dead Bug with Leg Raise:** 3 sets of 10 repetitions per side. Extend one leg straight up while maintaining lower back press and core engagement.
- **Cool-down:** Same as Week 1.

Workout 2: Stability & Power:

- **Warm-up:** Same as Week 1.

- **Side Plank with Reach & Overhead Press:** 3 sets of 10-12 repetitions per side. Hold a light weight and reach under your body while pressing overhead.
- **Weighted Russian Twist Walk:** 3 sets of 12 repetitions per side with medicine ball or dumbbell. Walk hands and weights to one side, perform a twist, and walk back.
- **Single-Leg Romanian Deadlift with Reach:** 3 sets of 10-12 repetitions per leg. Reach towards the ground as you lower the weight, maintaining a flat back and engaged core.
- **Hollow Body Hold with Leg Raises:** 3 sets of 30-second holds with alternate leg raises. Focus on core engagement and keeping your lower back pressed to the ground.
- **Cool-down:** Same as Week 1.

Workout 3: Core Blast with Progressions:

- **Warm-up:** Same as Week 1.
- **Russian Twist with Leg Raise:** 3 sets of 8-10 repetitions per side with light

weights. Raise one leg as you twist, challenging your core and balance.

- **Mountain Climbers with Torso Twist:** 3 sets of 30 seconds. Alternate bringing knees towards your chest while twisting your torso slightly to one side.
- **Plank Shoulder Taps:** 3 sets of 10-12 repetitions per side. In a plank position, tap your shoulder with your opposite hand, maintaining core engagement.
- **Side Plank with Hip Dips:** 3 sets of 10-12 repetitions per side. Lower your hips slightly while maintaining a side plank position.
- **Cool-down:** Same as Week 1.

Remember:

- Listen to your body and adjust weights or exercises as needed.
- Track your progress! Celebrate improvements and adjust workouts for continued challenge.
- Stay hydrated and fueled for optimal performance.

- Share your experiences and support fellow challengers in the community (if available).

Week 2 will test your limits, but remember, you're building a stronger, more defined core with each workout. Get ready to conquer Week 3 and unlock your core's true potential!

Week 3: Pushing Limits - Unleash Your Core Mastery!

Welcome to Week 3, challengers! Prepare to **push your limits, explore advanced variations, and experience the true power of the Russian Twist**. This week's workouts will **challenge your core strength, stability, and control** like never before. Embrace the burn, trust in your progress, and witness your core transformation accelerate!

Key Focus:

- Introducing advanced variations of the Russian Twist and other core exercises.
- Combining exercises for dynamic core challenges.
- Pushing your limits while maintaining proper form and safety.

Workout Structure:

This week you'll have three 35-minute workouts focusing on advanced variations and complex movements. Remember, **prioritize form over**

speed or heavier weights, and adjust exercises as needed.

Workout 1: Advanced Core Circuit:

- **Warm-up:** Same as Week 1 and 2, with additional dynamic stretches focusing on core and shoulders.
- **Hanging Russian Twist:** 3 sets of 10-12 repetitions per side. Hang from a pull-up bar and perform controlled twists. Modify with knee raises if needed.
- **Medicine Ball Slam Twist:** 3 sets of 10-12 repetitions per side. Slam a medicine ball to the ground as you twist, engaging core and upper body.
- **TRX Rollout with Twist:** 3 sets of 8-10 repetitions. Use TRX straps to perform a rollout while adding a torso twist at the end.
- **Anti-Rotation Press with Walkout:** 3 sets of 10-12 repetitions per side. Hold weights and resist rotation while walking your hands out to a plank and back.
- **Cool-down:** Same as Week 1 and 2.

Workout 2: Dynamic Core Flow:

- **Warm-up:** Same as Workout 1.
- **Russian Twist Walkout:** 3 sets of 10 repetitions per side. Walk hands and weights out to a plank, perform a twist, and walk back to center.
- **V-Ups:** 3 sets of 10-12 repetitions. Lie on your back, extend legs and torso simultaneously, engaging your core. Modify with crunches if needed.
- **Side Plank Hip Swivels:** 3 sets of 10 repetitions per side. Maintain a side plank and swivel your hips up and down, keeping your core engaged.
- **Plank Supermans:** 3 sets of 10-12 repetitions. In a plank position, alternate extending one arm and opposite leg, maintaining a flat back and engaged core.
- **Cool-down:** Same as Week 1 and 2.

Workout 3: Core & Strength Fusion:

- **Warm-up:** Same as Workout 1.

- **Weighted Russian Twist with Leg Raise and Reach:** 3 sets of 8-10 repetitions per side. Add weights, raise one leg, and reach your opposite hand towards the ground for an ultimate core challenge.
- **Squat to Press with Anti-Rotation:** 3 sets of 10-12 repetitions. Squat down, stand up while pressing weights overhead, and resist rotation with each movement.
- **Hanging Knee Raise Twist:** 3 sets of 10-12 repetitions per side. Hang from a pull-up bar, bring knees towards chest, and twist at the peak.
- **Dead Bug with Arm and Leg Reach:** 3 sets of 10 repetitions per side. Extend opposite arm and leg simultaneously, maintaining lower back press and core engagement.
- **Cool-down:** Same as Week 1 and 2.

Remember:

- This week is about intensity and exploration. You might need to modify exercises or decrease weights based on your fitness level.

- Track your progress and note down any modifications you make.
- Celebrate your achievements and stay motivated by sharing your journey with the community (if available).
- Listen to your body and prioritize proper form to avoid injury.

Week 3 will push you to your limits, but trust that you're building a stronger, more defined core with each rep. Embrace the challenge, conquer the advanced variations, and get ready to experience true core mastery in Week 4!

Week 4: Peak Performance - Celebrate Your Core Transformation!

Welcome to Week 4, challengers! It's time to **peak your performance, celebrate your transformation, and unleash the final burst of power in your core**. This week's workouts will **fine-tune your technique, test your strength, and leave you feeling empowered and proud of your achievements**.

Key Focus:

- Refining form and technique for all Russian Twist variations.
- Pushing your limits with peak performance challenges.
- Celebrating your progress and enjoying the rewards of your hard work.

Workout Structure:

This week you'll have three 30-minute workouts focusing on **peak performance exercises and a celebratory finale**. Remember, **prioritize form**

over speed or heavier weights, and adapt exercises as needed.

Workout 1: Peak Twist Technique:

- **Warm-up:** Same as Week 1 and 2, with additional focus on dynamic core and shoulder stretches.
- **Master the Classics:** 3 sets of 12-15 repetitions per side for each variation: bodyweight Russian Twist, weighted Russian Twist, Russian Twist with Leg Raise. Focus on perfect form and controlled movements.
- **Anti-Rotation Twists:** 3 sets of 10-12 repetitions per side. Choose 2-3 variations you enjoy (medicine ball, cable machine, band) and focus on resisting rotational forces while strengthening your core.
- **Plank Variations:** 3 sets of 30-second holds each. Choose 2-3 variations you enjoy (regular plank, side plank, hollow body hold) and focus on core engagement and proper form.
- **Cool-down:** Same as Week 1 and 2.

Workout 2: Peak Performance Challenge:

- **Warm-up:** Same as Workout 1.
- **Timed Russian Twist Circuit:** Perform each variation for 30 seconds straight, with minimal rest in between: hanging Russian Twist, medicine ball slam Twist, TRX rollout with Twist. Rest for 1 minute and repeat the circuit 2-3 times.
- **AMRAP Core Blast:** Do as many reps as possible (AMRAP) of each exercise for 1 minute each: side plank hip swivels, V-ups, plank supermans. Rest for 30 seconds and repeat the circuit 2-3 times.
- **Superset Challenge:** Combine 2 core exercises with minimal rest for intense challenge: squat to press with anti-rotation + hanging knee raise twist, dead bug with arm and leg reach + weighted Russian Twist with leg raise and reach. Repeat each superset 3 times with 30 seconds rest in between.
- **Cool-down:** Same as Week 1 and 2.

Workout 3: Celebration Finale:

- **Warm-up:** Light cardio and dynamic stretches.
- **Create Your Own Core Flow:** Design a 20-minute flow using your favorite Russian Twist variations, core exercises, and progressions from this challenge. Focus on fun, celebrate your progress, and enjoy the final workout!
- **Cool-down:** Deep static stretches focusing on core, back, and legs.
- **Celebration Time!** Take a moment to reflect on your journey, the challenges you conquered, and the stronger, more defined core you built. Share your achievements with the community (if available), reward yourself for your hard work, and be proud of your transformation!

Remember:

- This week is about celebrating your journey and showcasing your peak performance. Listen to your body and adjust exercises as needed.

- Share your final workout flow and achievements with the community (if available) and inspire others.
- Don't stop moving! Maintain an active lifestyle, incorporate core exercises into your routine, and continue your core transformation journey.

Congratulations on completing the 4-week Russian Twist Challenge! You've built a stronger, more defined core, increased your strength and endurance, and proven your dedication to fitness. Remember, this is just the beginning! Keep moving, keep challenging yourself, and continue sculpting your dream core!

Chapter 6

Fueling Your Core - Rest, Recovery, and Nutrition for Peak Performance

Building a sculpted core isn't just about intense workouts; it's about nurturing your body with **rest, recovery, and proper nutrition**. This chapter equips you with the knowledge to optimize these essential elements, ensuring your efforts translate into **maximum results and a sustainable transformation**.

Rest & Recovery:

- **Listen to your body:** It craves rest after challenging workouts. Schedule rest days (at least 1-2 per week) and listen to fatigue cues during workouts. Pushing through pain can lead to injury.
- **Active recovery:** Light activities like walking, yoga, or swimming promote blood flow and aid muscle repair. Choose

activities you enjoy to avoid feeling burnt
out.

- **Sleep:** Aim for 7-8 hours of quality sleep
  each night. Sleep is crucial for muscle
  repair, hormone regulation, and overall
  recovery.
- **Stretching and foam rolling:** Regularly
  stretch your core muscles and use a foam
  roller to release tension and improve
  flexibility. This can also help prevent
  injuries.

Nutrition:

- **Eat for your goals:** Focus on consuming
  whole, unprocessed foods rich in protein,
  healthy fats, and complex carbohydrates.
  These nutrients provide the building
  blocks for muscle growth and energy to
  fuel your workouts.
- **Protein is king:** Aim for 0.8-1 gram of
  protein per pound of body weight daily to
  support muscle repair and growth. Lean
  protein sources like chicken, fish, beans,
  and tofu are excellent choices.

- **Healthy fats are your friends:** Include healthy fats like avocados, nuts, and olive oil in your diet. These fats provide essential nutrients and contribute to satiety, helping you manage calorie intake.
- **Stay hydrated:** Drink plenty of water throughout the day, especially before, during, and after workouts. Hydration is crucial for optimal performance and recovery.
- **Limit processed foods:** Sugary drinks, processed snacks, and excessive saturated and trans fats can hinder your progress. Opt for whole, unprocessed foods whenever possible.
- **Fuel your workouts:** Have a light, pre-workout snack rich in complex carbohydrates and protein to provide sustained energy. After your workout, opt for a recovery meal or snack with protein and carbohydrates to replenish glycogen stores and aid muscle repair.

Remember:

- Consistency is key. Sticking to a healthy diet and incorporating rest and recovery strategies consistently will yield better results than crash diets or sporadic efforts.
- Consult a registered dietitian or nutritionist for personalized guidance tailored to your specific needs and goals.
- Enjoy your food! Choose a variety of healthy options that you find delicious and satisfying to make long-term adherence easier.

By prioritizing rest, recovery, and proper nutrition alongside your challenging workouts, you'll create the perfect environment for your core to transform, reach its full potential, and propel you towards achieving your fitness goals!

This chapter concludes your personalized core transformation guide. Remember, consistency, dedication, and smart choices are the keys to success. Embrace the journey, celebrate your progress, and continue sculpting your dream core!

Chapter 7

Conquering Your Core Transformation: Tracking Progress & Staying Motivated

This final chapter equips you with essential tools to **track your progress** and **stay motivated** throughout your core transformation journey. Remember, visible changes may take time, but consistently monitoring your progress and fostering a positive mindset are key to reaching your goals.

Tracking Progress:

- **Log your workouts:** Record exercises, sets, reps, weights used, and any modifications made. This helps you monitor progress, identify areas for improvement, and adjust your workouts accordingly.
- **Progress photos:** Take photos at the beginning, middle, and end of the

challenge to visually track changes in body composition. Remember, focus on overall health and well-being, not just aesthetics.

- **Measurements:** Track your body measurements (waist, hips, etc.) to assess progress beyond the scale. Measurements can fluctuate, so combine them with other tracking methods for a holistic picture.
- **Strength gains:** Track the weight you lift or the number of reps you can perform for specific exercises. This helps you measure your increasing strength and adjust workouts for continued progress.
- **Performance and endurance:** Monitor changes in your performance during exercises like planks or Russian Twists. Can you hold them longer or perform more reps? Celebrate these improvements!

Staying Motivated:

- **Set realistic goals:** Start with small, achievable goals and gradually progress.

Celebrate each milestone to maintain momentum.

- **Find a workout buddy:** Partnering with someone can boost accountability, provide support, and make workouts more enjoyable.
- **Join a community:** Connect with others on a similar journey through online forums or fitness groups. Share experiences, motivate each other, and celebrate successes together.
- **Reward yourself:** Celebrate milestones and achievements with non-food rewards like a relaxing activity or a new workout outfit. This reinforces positive behaviors and keeps you engaged.
- **Focus on progress, not perfection:** Everyone experiences setbacks. Don't get discouraged; learn from them, adjust your approach, and keep moving forward.
- **Visualize your goals:** Create a vision board or write down your goals and aspirations. Regularly visualizing your

desired outcome can fuel your motivation
and keep you focused.

- **Enjoy the process:** Find activities within
the challenge that you enjoy. Exercise
shouldn't feel like a chore; incorporate fun
and variety to keep things interesting.
- **Remember your "why":** Remind
yourself why you started this journey.
Reconnecting with your initial
motivations can rekindle your passion and
commitment.

Remember:

- Tracking progress is a valuable tool, but
avoid obsessing over it. Focus on
consistency, effort, and enjoying the
journey.
- Motivation fluctuates. Be kind to yourself,
accept setbacks, and don't be afraid to
adjust your approach to stay on track.
- Celebrate every victory, big or small.
Recognizing your progress fuels your
motivation and keeps you moving towards
your goals.

Chapter 8

Beyond the Challenge - Integrate the Russian Twist into Your Fitness Routine

Congratulations on completing the 4-week Russian Twist Challenge! You've built a stronger, more defined core, pushed your limits, and experienced the power of consistency. While the challenge may be over, your core transformation journey doesn't have to end there. Let's explore how to **seamlessly integrate the Russian Twist into your long-term fitness routine**:

Benefits of Ongoing Integration:

- **Maintain core strength and stability:** A strong core supports proper posture, improves balance, and enhances performance in other exercises.
- **Prevent injuries:** A strong core helps protect your spine and reduce the risk of

injuries during daily activities and other
workouts.

- **Boost metabolism:** Core exercises like
  the Russian Twist engage multiple muscle
  groups, potentially leading to a slightly
  increased calorie burn.
- **Improve athletic performance:** Core
  strength is crucial for various sports and
  activities, enhancing power, agility, and
  overall performance.

Integration Strategies:

- **Weekly incorporation:** Aim for 2-3
  Russian Twist sessions per week,
  incorporating variations and progressions
  from the challenge, or exploring new
  variations found online or in fitness apps.
- **Warm-up or cool-down addition:**
  Include the Russian Twist as a warm-up
  exercise to activate your core before your
  main workout, or use it as a cool-down
  exercise to stretch and strengthen your
  core muscles.

- **Circuit training integration:** Combine the Russian Twist with other bodyweight or weighted exercises for a dynamic and challenging circuit workout.
- **Cross-training inclusion:** If you participate in other sports or activities, consider incorporating the Russian Twist or similar core exercises into your training routine to improve overall performance.

Advanced Variations & Tips:

- **Weighted variations:** As you progress, add weights (medicine balls, dumbbells) to increase the challenge and target deeper core muscles.
- **Unstable surfaces:** Perform the Russian Twist on an exercise ball or BOSU ball for an extra balance and core stability challenge.
- **Timed sets:** Challenge yourself with timed sets, aiming for a specific number of repetitions within a set time frame.
- **Circuit combinations:** Experiment with different exercise combinations and circuit

structures to keep your workouts fresh and engaging.

Remember:

- **Listen to your body:** Adjust the intensity, frequency, and variations of the Russian Twist based on your fitness level and goals.
- **Prioritize proper form:** Focus on controlled movements and engage your core muscles throughout the exercise to avoid injury.
- **Combine with a balanced routine:** The Russian Twist is a valuable tool, but don't neglect other aspects of fitness like cardiovascular exercise, strength training, and flexibility.
- **Have fun and be creative:** Explore different variations, experiment with circuits, and find ways to make the Russian Twist enjoyable to keep you motivated in the long run.

By integrating the Russian Twist into your ongoing fitness routine, you'll maintain your core strength, unlock further progress, and experience the lasting benefits of a strong and defined core. Remember, your fitness journey is ongoing, so embrace the challenge, stay active, and keep sculpting your best self!

Chapter 9

Pushing Your Limits - Advanced Variations and Training Techniques

Congratulations on conquering the Russian Twist Challenge and achieving a stronger, more defined core! But your journey doesn't have to end there. For those seeking an even greater challenge and further core development, this chapter dives into **advanced variations and training techniques** to push your limits and unlock new levels of core strength and control.

Advanced Variations:

- **Weighted Russian Twist with Leg Variations:**
    - **Russian Twist with Plate Hold:** Hold a weight plate close to your chest while performing the twist for added upper body challenge.

- **Single-Leg Russian Twist with Kettlebell:** Perform the twist while balancing on one leg and holding a kettlebell in the opposite hand.
  - **Weighted Russian Twist with Leg Raise:** Add a leg raise at the peak of the twist, holding a weight in the raised leg for an ultimate core and balance challenge.
- **Unstable Surface Variations:**
  - **Swiss Ball Russian Twist:** Perform the twist while seated on a Swiss ball, engaging your core to maintain stability.
  - **BOSU Ball Russian Twist:** Increase the instability by performing the twist on a BOSU ball, requiring constant core activation for balance.
  - **Foam Roller Russian Twist:** Add a foam roller under your lower back for an extra core and spine stabilization challenge.
- **Dynamic & Combination Variations:**

- **Medicine Ball Slam Twist:** Slam a
  medicine ball to the ground as you
  twist, combining power and core
  engagement.
- **TRX Rollout with Twist:** Use
  TRX straps to perform a rollout
  while adding a torso twist at the end
  for a dynamic core blast.
- **Hanging Windmill:** Hang from a
  pull-up bar and perform controlled
  windmill rotations, challenging
  your core and grip strength.

Training Techniques:

- **Supersets & Circuits:** Combine the
  Russian Twist with other core exercises
  (planks, side planks, V-ups) in supersets
  or circuits for an intense core workout.
- **Drop Sets & AMRAPs:** Increase the
  intensity by reducing weight or reps
  throughout a set (drop sets) or aiming for
  as many reps as possible within a set time
  frame (AMRAPs).

- **Tempo Variations:** Slow down the movement (slow tempo) to increase muscle tension and time under tension, or speed up the movement (fast tempo) for an agility and power challenge.
- **Isometric Holds:** Hold the Russian Twist at the peak of the contraction for a set time (e.g., 30 seconds) to build isometric strength and core endurance.

Important Tips:

- **Always prioritize proper form over heavier weights or faster speeds.** Incorrect form can lead to injury.
- **Warm up properly before training and cool down afterwards.**
- **Listen to your body and take rest days when needed.**
- **Combine advanced variations with bodyweight exercises to maintain balance and prevent overuse injuries.**
- **Seek guidance from a certified personal trainer if you have any concerns or limitations.**

Remember:

By incorporating these advanced variations and training techniques, you can continue to challenge your core, unlock new levels of strength and control, and keep your core transformation journey exciting and progressive. However, always prioritize safety, listen to your body, and enjoy the process of pushing your limits and achieving your fitness goals!

Chapter 10

Building a Strong Core for Overall Fitness and Performance

The journey to a sculpted core isn't just about aesthetics; it's about building a strong foundation for **overall fitness and performance**. A strong core empowers you to move with **confidence, stability, and power**, enhancing your experiences in various aspects of life:

Improved Everyday Activities:

- **Enhanced posture and reduced back pain:** A strong core supports your spine, improves posture, and prevents back pain caused by poor alignment or weak muscles.
- **Increased balance and coordination:** Core strength contributes to better balance and coordination, leading to safer and

more confident movement in daily activities.

- **Greater functional strength:** Lifting groceries, playing with kids, or climbing stairs become easier and less strenuous with a strong core.

Boosting Athletic Performance:

- **Power and explosiveness:** Strong core muscles generate power for various movements, improving your performance in running, jumping, throwing, and other athletic activities.
- **Enhanced stability and injury prevention:** A strong core stabilizes your body during movements, reducing the risk of injuries caused by imbalances or weak core muscles.
- **Improved efficiency and endurance:** Core strength contributes to efficient energy use and better endurance, allowing you to perform for longer and at a higher intensity.

Benefits Beyond Movement:

- **Improved breathing and respiratory function:** Core muscles support your diaphragm and enhance efficient breathing, impacting overall health and well-being.
- **Enhanced mental well-being:** Physical activity, including core training, releases endorphins and reduces stress, contributing to positive mental health.
- **Increased confidence and self-esteem:** Achieving fitness goals and building a strong core can boost your confidence and self-esteem, positively impacting various aspects of your life.

Remember:

- **A strong core is the foundation for a healthy and active lifestyle.**
- **Core training is not just about crunches and sit-ups; it involves various exercises targeting different core muscles.**

- **Consistency is key! Regular core training, even just a few minutes daily, can significantly impact your overall fitness and well-being.**

Chapter 11

Core Training Myths Debunked - Separating Fact from Fiction

Building a strong core is a journey filled with information and advice, but not all of it is accurate. This chapter tackles some **common core training myths** to help you separate fact from fiction and optimize your core transformation journey:

Myth 1: Crunches are the best core exercise.

Fact: While crunches can activate some core muscles, they primarily target the upper abs and neglect other crucial core areas. A well-rounded core workout incorporates exercises targeting various muscle groups, including planks, side planks, anti-rotation exercises, and Russian Twists.

Myth 2: Spot reduction is possible with core exercises.

Fact: Unfortunately, you cannot target specific fat loss through exercise alone. While core exercises can strengthen and define your core muscles, they won't necessarily burn fat from your belly specifically. Overall balanced diet and exercise contribute to healthy fat loss throughout the body.

Myth 3: Pain during core exercises is normal.

Fact: While some muscle soreness is expected after challenging workouts, sharp pain is not a sign of progress. It could indicate improper form, overuse, or an underlying injury. Always prioritize proper form and stop if you experience pain.

Myth 4: Six-pack abs are the only sign of a strong core.

Fact: While visible abs are aesthetically pleasing, they don't necessarily equate to a strong core. A strong core is about overall functionality, stability, and power, not just aesthetics. Focus on building a strong core foundation, and visible abs may follow as a result of consistent training and healthy habits.

Myth 5: You need expensive equipment for effective core training.

Fact: You can achieve a strong core with minimal or no equipment. Bodyweight exercises like planks, V-ups, and bird-dogs are highly effective. As you progress, consider using affordable tools like medicine balls, resistance bands, or exercise balls for added challenge and variety.

Remember:

- **Critical thinking is key:** Don't blindly accept every piece of advice you hear. Research, consult experts, and listen to your body.
- **Focus on form over intensity:** Prioritize proper form to avoid injuries and maximize results.

- **Consistency is crucial:** Regular core training, even for short periods, is more effective than sporadic intense workouts.
- **Enjoy the process:** Find core exercises you enjoy to make them sustainable and maintain motivation.

By debunking these common myths and focusing on evidence-based practices, you can approach your core training journey with confidence and achieve your desired results. Remember, a strong core is not just about aesthetics; it's an investment in your overall health, performance, and well-being. So, stay informed, stay motivated, and keep sculpting your strongest, healthiest self!

Conclusion

Congratulations! You've reached the final chapter of your personalized core transformation guide. By incorporating the knowledge, strategies, and workouts throughout this guide, you've built a stronger, more defined core, pushed your limits, and experienced the power of dedication and consistency. However, the journey doesn't end here. This chapter provides key tips to **maintain your core transformation** and continue building upon your achievements:

Maintaining Motivation:

- **Celebrate your progress:** Take time to reflect on how far you've come. Celebrate milestones, big and small, to stay motivated and appreciate your efforts.
- **Set new goals:** Keep challenging yourself with new goals, whether it's mastering an advanced variation, increasing workout intensity, or trying a new core training program.

- **Find enjoyment:** Choose core exercises you enjoy and incorporate activities you find fun. Exercise shouldn't feel like a chore; make it something you look forward to.
- **Track your progress:** Continue tracking your workouts and progress in a way that motivates you. Seeing measurable results fuels your dedication and reinforces positive behaviors.
- **Find a support system:** Surround yourself with supportive friends, family, or online communities who encourage your fitness journey and celebrate your victories.

Sustainable Practices:

- **Incorporate core training into your routine:** Dedicate 2-3 sessions per week to core exercises, integrating them into your existing fitness routine or as standalone workouts.
- **Focus on functional movements:** Don't just chase aesthetics; choose core

exercises that translate into improved functionality and performance in daily activities or specific sports.

- **Prioritize proper form:** Always prioritize proper form over heavier weights or faster speeds to avoid injury and maximize long-term benefits.
- **Listen to your body:** Take rest days when needed, adjust exercises based on your limitations, and don't push through pain.
- **Fuel your body right:** Maintain a healthy diet that supports your fitness goals and provides essential nutrients for optimal performance and recovery.

Expanding Your Horizons:

- **Explore new exercises:** Continuously discover new core exercises and variations to keep your workouts fresh and challenging.
- **Try different training methods:** Experiment with supersets, circuits, HIIT workouts, or bodyweight challenges to

keep your core engaged and challenged in different ways.

- **Seek professional guidance:** Consider consulting a certified personal trainer for personalized workout plans, form checks, and additional guidance based on your specific needs and goals.
- **Challenge yourself in other areas:** Branch out and explore other fitness activities like yoga, Pilates, or dance, which can further enhance your core strength and flexibility.

Remember:

Building a strong, healthy core is a lifelong journey, not a sprint. By incorporating these tips and maintaining a consistent approach, you can sustain your core transformation, unlock new levels of strength and performance, and continue reaping the benefits of a strong core in all aspects of your life. Embrace the journey, celebrate your progress, and keep empowering yourself with a strong, confident core!

Sample Warm-up and Cool-down Routines:

Warm-up (5-10 minutes):

Focus: Gradually increase heart rate, activate core muscles, and prepare for exercise.

Cardio:

- **Light jog:** 3-5 minutes at a comfortable pace.
- **Jumping jacks:** 2 sets of 15-20 reps.
- **High knees:** 2 sets of 20 reps per leg.
- **Butt kicks:** 2 sets of 20 reps per leg.

Dynamic stretches:

- **Arm circles:** Forward and backward, 10 reps each direction.
- **Torso twists:** Gentle rotations, 10 reps each direction.
- **Leg swings:** Front and back, 10 reps each direction.
- **Walking lunges:** 10-15 reps per leg.
- **Side lunges:** 10-15 reps per leg.

Core activation:

- **Bird-dogs:** 10 reps per side.
- **Dead bugs:** 10 reps per side.
- **Plank:** 30-second hold.

Cool-down (5-10 minutes):

Focus: Gradually decrease heart rate, cool down muscles, and improve flexibility.

Cardio:

- **Walking:** 3-5 minutes at a leisurely pace.

Static stretches:

- **Hamstring stretch:** Sit and reach towards your toes, hold for 30 seconds.
- **Quad stretch:** Stand and hold your ankle behind you, pulling your heel towards your buttocks, hold for 30 seconds.
- **Calf stretch:** Lean against a wall with one leg forward and one leg back, push your heel down, hold for 30 seconds per leg.

- **Chest stretch:** Clasp your hands behind your back and gently push your chest forward, hold for 30 seconds.
- **Arm stretches:** Overhead reach, tricep stretch, and bicep stretch, hold each for 30 seconds.

Remember:

- These are just samples, adjust the exercises and duration based on your fitness level and workout intensity.
- Listen to your body and modify exercises as needed.
- Breathe deeply and slowly throughout the warm-up and cool-down.

I hope this helps!

Bonus

Printable Workout Logs and Trackers:

Here are some options for printable workout logs and trackers you can use to monitor your progress throughout your core transformation journey:

Basic Workout Log:

This is a simple template with space to record the date, exercise, sets, reps, weight (if applicable), and any notes:

https://docs.google.com/spreadsheets/d/1Rh0EI7YA-scykp6BnQzEpqRYZPrIwhNs7qTwWpNsnlM/edit?usp=drivesdk

Link for workout log sheet

Advanced Workout Log:

This template includes additional columns for tracking rest time, perceived exertion (e.g., RPE scale), and modifications:

https://docs.google.com/spreadsheets/d/1N3kM
OgWPnuEPeprcG8-TpN9BkrJ1gNJSyhOHa_hh
90M/edit?usp=drivesdk

Weekly Core Tracker:

This template allows you to track your core
workouts throughout the week, with space for
logging specific exercises and variations:

https://docs.google.com/spreadsheets/d/1tZXRS
dhu-y9YnYhOzpN6wnZRh3f95TkTKfTNb1n05
gE/edit?usp=drivesdk

Progress Tracker:

This template helps you monitor your progress over time by recording measurements like body weight, waist circumference, and body fat percentage:

https://docs.google.com/spreadsheets/d/1XMUF HKGn2Qx9omUt8nGeejy93e2dzK7zrCaQsZVtf tk/edit?usp=drivesdk

Tips:

- Choose a template that fits your needs and preferences.
- Print them on cardstock or laminate them for durability.
- Keep them in a binder or folder for easy access.
- Decorate them or add personal touches to make them more fun.

- Be consistent with your tracking for accurate results.

Video tutorial link

https://screenpal.com/watch/cZnQY1VdvZu

You've reached the culmination of your Core Transformation Challenge! Embarking on this journey, you mastered the Russian Twist, explored its variations, and pushed your limits further than you imagined. But remember, this **isn't an ending, it's a beginning**.

This challenge was your catalyst, igniting the spark of a stronger, more confident you. You've built a foundation of core strength, sculpted definition, and experienced the power of dedication. But true transformation extends beyond aesthetics. It's about resilience, empowerment, and carrying that core strength into every aspect of your life.

Here are some takeaways to remember as you move forward:

- **Consistency is key:** Short bursts of effort are valuable, but lasting results come from regular practice. Integrate core training into your routine, even for 10 minutes daily, and witness the cumulative impact.

- **Explore and adapt:** Don't get stuck in a rut. Explore new variations, discover different training methods, and keep your workouts fresh and engaging.
- **Listen to your body:** It whispers before it screams. Respect your limitations, prioritize proper form, and take rest when needed. Injuries can derail your progress, so listen to your body's wisdom.
- **Celebrate progress, not perfection:** Focus on how far you've come, not how far you have to go. Every rep, every drop of sweat is a victory. Celebrate milestones, big and small, to stay motivated.
- **Fuel your body:** You can't out-train a bad diet. Nourish your body with wholesome foods to optimize performance, recovery, and overall well-being.
- **Embrace the journey:** This is not just about achieving a six-pack; it's about embracing a healthier, happier you. Find joy in movement, connect with

like-minded individuals, and let the
journey itself be your reward.

Remember, your core is more than just muscles;
it's the center of your strength, stability, and
confidence. Carry that newfound power with
you, continue exploring your potential, and keep
sculpting your best self - a self empowered by a
strong, resilient core.

Congratulations on embarking on this transformative journey. May your core strength continue to guide you towards achieving your goals and living life to the fullest!